# Choices

Elaine Lawrence Wynn, Ph.D.

iUniverse, Inc.
Bloomington

*iUniverse*
*1663 Liberty Drive*
*Bloomington, IN 47403*

*This publication is intended to provide educational and informative material on the subject matter covered. In no way should it be considered as offering medical advice. It is written with the understanding that the author is not engaged in rendering professional services in the book. If you experience any symptoms described in this book, do not assume it is because of the subject matter being discussed. Your symptoms may be caused by other health conditions. If you experience any one of them, see your physician. The author specifically disclaims any responsibility for any liability, loss, or risk, personal or otherwise, which is incurred as a consequence, directly or indirectly, of the use and application of any of the contents of this book.*

*Because of the dynamic nature of the Internet, any Web addresses or links contained in this book may have changed since publication and may no longer be valid. The views expressed in this work are solely those of the author and do not necessarily reflect the views of the publisher, and the publisher hereby disclaims any responsibility for them.*

*ISBN: 978-1-4502-6205-7 (sc)*
*ISBN: 978-1-4502-6206-4 (ebook)*

*Printed in the United States of America*

*iUniverse rev. date: 11/22/2010*

# Dedication

*Here's to Your Health!!*

# Acknowledgments

*The following people are owed my deepest thanks for their inspiring commitment to the creation of this book:*

*First, to my husband Raymond for your love and dedication.*

*Second, to my parents, Dorothy and Eddie Lawrence, for helping me to realize that breaking generational bondages was necessary and that I could take control of my health and not suffer ailments of our ancestors.*

*Third, to my sons, Terrance and Courtney for pushing me to "exercise," "go to the gym," and "work out." Your persistence turned a dreaded daily task into a simple pleasure that I now look forward to. Both of you have been a great blessing and delight.*

*And finally to my audience, thank you for your support.*

# Preface

*I awaken one morning to an epiphany – one of those moments when the light bulb goes off and you finally see the whole picture. Then you have a really novel idea. I realized that high blood pressure, heart disease, diabetes, strokes, cancer and negative people were all around me. They were bombarding our existence like a thief in the night with the sole purpose of destroying us. Generation after generation of people in my family had succumbed to the hands of this deadly force. Then after two battles of cancer in my immediate family, my thought to myself was, "This is insane." But what was more enlightening was realizing that I was following the same unhealthy eating habits and practices as my ancestors and expecting not to suffer the same type of aliments. How insane (doing the same thing over and over again and expecting a different result) was that? At that point, I decided I was not going down without a fight. My mindset had to be transformed; generational bondages had to be broken; positive energy had to consume me; and my health had to improve because a lot of the practices that I had been taught and adapted through the years about eating and caring for my health obviously were not working. The statistics spoke for themselves time and time again as one family member after another was having massive heart attacks or being diagnosed with illnesses that could have been prevented if THEY HAD ONLY KNOWN...*

*Well, I consider myself a pretty intelligent person so the madness had to stop here. I was open to new ideas. In fact, I looked for them. The CHOICE was mine. Living a healthy lifestyle was my preference and I'm in control and winning the battle. So, how's your health? After reading this book you will be empowered to make adjustments that put you on the road to living a healthier lifestyle as well.*

You want real talk?

Here's real talk…

There is something about you that definitely needs to CHANGE.

Jennie Craig, South Beach, or Atkins…the kind of diet does not matter if you are not going to discipline yourself enough to change your lifestyle. Millions of dollars are spent each year in the dieting industry. Teenagers to great great-grandparents, male and female participate in this fetish which is expensive and very time consuming. Many people consistently exercise day after day; refuse to eat certain foods because of the calorie intake; and lose a few pounds to no avail (they gain more weight than they had before they started dieting a few months later). As a result, many of them try another diet. It is a vicious cycle. What they fail to realize is that in order to lose weight they must take in fewer calories than they burn, apart from the amount of exercise they do and that eating right requires making better food choices, consistency and discipline. Eating healthier must become a way of life.

When the word diet is mentioned, we tend to immediately think a regime of limited food or drink taken in by a person in order to lose weight. We are inclined to dismiss the fact that when a person says "diet" he (she) could be referring to his (her) intake of food and beverages on a daily basis and that it has nothing to do with losing unwanted inches from around the waistline. It is from the latter viewpoint that this book is written. Allow me to sketch an image in your mind of daily activities of a person that has chosen to live a healthier lifestyle. You will be faced with many of the same choices once you begin your journey to a better way of life.

As I was reading in an office lobby one day, a man said to me, "Every time I see you, there is a book in your hand and you're reading. Why is that?" I said to him then, as I say to you now, I am a firm believer that knowledge is power and we must know how to activate that power inside and outside of ourselves in order to be successful. I believe that people are destroyed for a lack of knowledge. Therefore, we must not only increase our knowledge base everyday but also apply to our lives noteworthy principles that we learn in order to become the best person that we can be. It is imperative that we realize, as the old adage goes, "I'm a work in progress."

Our bodies are very similar to relationships. You get out of them what you put into them. And the condition of the relationship is often a reflection of one's self. Likewise, you are what you eat. It is a very simple principle of sowing and reaping. If you lack discipline, eat a lot of junk foods, desserts, pastries, bad fat, drink inadequate amounts of water and fail to exercise (just to name a few things), you are setting yourself up for a range of illnesses, from as simple as the common cold to more serious diseases. On the other hand, if you eat healthy, exercise, drink adequate amounts of water, and do what you should do for your well-being, you are increasing the level of satisfaction you have within yourself and promoting longevity. Besides, at the end of the day, longevity has a lot more to do with your choices than with your DNA and being lucky.

Now, before describing a typical day in the life of a person who has chosen to live a healthier lifestyle, let's discuss six prerequisites that must be worked through in order for you to be successful in your new daily routine. Each prerequisite has more than one task associated with it which requires different types of introspection.

# # 1    Examine Your Mindset

The first prerequisite towards developing a healthy lifestyle is examining your mindset or how you think. You have to want to change and become a better, healthier person before you can successfully change anything in your life. The decision must be yours. No one can make you do anything that you do not want to do. My wanting you to be healthy is not going to make that happen unless that's your choice. The desire and drive must come from within you. This is significant because a person's physical health is often a reflection of their emotional and mental health. That's why a positive attitude speaks volumes about a person. Your transformation to a healthier lifestyle must begin in your mind. The mind is a very powerful instrument. For it is within the mind that all perception (which will eventually become your reality) is created. Living healthier must become a lifestyle and you have to work at it every day understanding that your ability to succeed depends upon your patient endurance and humility.

Have you ever noticed that people with negative attitudes are always complaining? From health issues to anything else in life they can possibly find to say something derogatory about, the list is endless. It would appear that their happiness is contingent upon seeing how miserable they can actually be or cause you to become. And why they always feel compelled to share their morbid thoughts with everyone they come in contact with is truly beyond comprehension. What they fail to realize is that complaining only forces a person to focus more on the undesirable circumstance. As a result, negative people can deplete your positive energy right out of you if you are not careful and mature in your thought process. In this context, being mature in your thought process means that you, a person living a healthy lifestyle, are able to recognize negative forces coming at you and you have the ability to effectively deflect them. This ability requires discernment in predicting where a conversation is headed and steering it into another direction or disarming it completely. For some people, this type of assertiveness takes a lot of practice. Therefore, at this early stage to acquiring a positive mental attitude, deliberately avoid negative people and people that gossip. Who is conveying the negative message or the juicy gossip is irrelevant. Stay away from them. This may mean avoiding conversations with family members, girlfriends, buddies, co-workers or even your neighbors. And if you have a negative spouse or significant other, it is your responsibility to discuss with him (her) how you have decided to transform your lifestyle and lovingly point out to him (her) the negativity and how it will effect you during the process of change. Ask him (her) to not display that behavior around you and if he (she) would work on getting rid of that type of mindset as well. Perhaps the two of you can work together and agree to gently bring to each other's attention when one of you hears the other speaking negatively. Look at it like this, your association with people who are negative or people that gossip can be compared to a person continuously breathing in carbon monoxide and believing that it won't kill him. Nothing could be further from the truth.

Protect your mind and be very selective about the information that you allow yourself to process. Another area that you will need to examine is the music you listen to. Determine what the lyrics of songs are really saying because music has a way of penetrating the mind, emotions and heart of those that indulge. If you don't agree with the lyrics, don't sing the song. It's not enough that the rhythm or beat sounds good. Today, the lyrics of many popular songs advocate behaviors that are absolutely demoralizing to man and the more you repeat and think about those things, the more they will become a part of you whether you want them to or not.

The same is true for movies and television shows. Evaluate the messages that their previews convey. Then develop a viewing criterion for yourself. Is the show demonstrating morals and ethics that you support? Is the language toxic? What seeds of information are you planting in your mind if you watch the show? Viewing criterion is so important because if you fail to establish your viewing standards, movie and television producers will create one for you. That is too great of a risk that could lead to devastating consequences. Negative thoughts and messages simply cannot be allowed to hover around in your mind and become a part of your thought process if you are serious about living a healthier lifestyle.

In fact, now is also the occasion to assess your relationships. There will be times on this journey when you will not be able to associate with people you have been very close to because their negative energy will hinder you from accomplishing your goal which is to become a healthier person. People that are important to you will have to be considered in terms similar to insurance, something that you must have but may not utilize at the moment. Are they assets or liabilities toward you accomplishing your goal of living a healthier lifestyle? This is your moment in time when you must make difficult but honest decisions regarding relationships in your life. Ask yourself whether significant others are positive people? Do they encourage you to be at the top of your game? Are they making advances in their own lives? When the odds are against you, do they offer an encouraging word or do they join in the pity party? Do they believe in you as a person and what you are trying to achieve in life? How do they respond when you are successful? When they see you getting ready to run into a brick wall, what is their response? Do they help you avoid a crisis or do they allow you to run right into it? What does your association with them add to you as a person? Do their good qualities outweigh the negative attributes? What type of affect do they have on you? How do you find yourself behaving when you are around them? Can you be yourself? Make a deliberate effort to minimize or eliminate contact with all liabilities at this time in your life.

It is also important to listen to and carefully evaluate what others are telling you about people in your life when they truly have your best interest in mind. Now of course, you cannot believe everything people say but when more than one person is saying the same thing (that you should not be involved with a particular person; or that a person does not have your best interest at heart) you need to listen and respond appropriately. It is unfortunate that sometimes we are so close to situations that we cannot see the true motives of some people or who they really are. However, it is at this point that you need to release yourself of people who can be considered harmful baggage – people who your association with causes you unduly hurt, pain, and stress. Don't be afraid to let them go. You cannot remain in bondage to people. Sometimes loving a person does not mean holding on to them; it means you letting them be free; or just letting them be. And drama queens should not be the type of people you allow in your social circle. Instead, find and make new acquaintances with individuals that complete who you are as a person and who you are striving to become. Discover your purpose in life. Why were you created? Then identify someone worthy of imitating who has already achieved the kind of goals that you want to accomplish. Study that person's positive attributes, strategies, and principles; learn from them and empower yourself.

As you move forward in making better choices for your life and experience the results, you will quickly develop strategies to keep you focused on what's best for you because you will love what you see in yourself and how you feel. Expect to have to make difficult choices in order to remain on course and be productive. In fact, an enormous part of your success will depend on the words you speak during this process. Therefore, guard your mouth and always choose carefully the words you communicate. Make no corrupt statements. Allow your conversation to demonstrate kindness to those that are listening to you. Develop a habit of looking for something good in every situation and all people. Think about this. You have the power to speak life or death into any situation; to build up a person or circumstance or tare it down. And regardless of your choice, it will revert back to the principle of sowing and reaping.

**The first prerequisite towards developing a healthy lifestyle is examining your mindset or how you think.**

- What parts of this prerequisite do you need to incorporate in your life in order to live a healthier lifestyle?

- How will you achieve this goal?

- By when do you want to achieve this goal?

- What obstacles can be expected?

- What are the solutions to the obstacles?

# # 2  You Will Have What You Say

The second prerequisite and one of the most powerful realizations you can have during this stage of conversion to a healthier lifestyle is to understand the notion of "you will have what you say." Therefore, it is imperative for you to develop a routine of reciting positive statements about your relationships, health, lifestyle, employment, and yourself (all facets of your life) several times each day. Words satisfy the soul just as food satisfies the stomach and those who love to talk will experience the consequences. For the tongue can destroy or nourish life. Therefore, if it is your desire to obtain a certain economic level, then state, "My economic level is increasing," and put into action what is necessary to accomplish that goal. Affirmations and action go hand-in-hand. It does no good to have one without the other. You can make positive statements all day but if you fail to implement a corresponding action to bring to fruition what you are saying and believing, nothing will happen. When you sit on the "stool of do nothing" you get nothing. You must make your way prosperous. Otherwise, your life will be ineffective with no results. Again it reverts back to the simple principle of sewing and reaping. By making affirmations you are training yourself to speak life into your own situations and forcing yourself to examine the positive aspects of your world that you are creating. Only after seeing yourself in a more positive perspective will you have the ability to observe the difference in your perceptions of and responses to people and situations as they occur in your life. You will find yourself being a positive agent of change and displaying a level of self confidence that will allow your aura to become contagious.

**The second prerequisite to living a healthier lifestyle is to realize that you will have what you say so recite positive statements about yourself several times each day.**

- Write several positive statements about yourself, your relationships, health, lifestyle, employment etc. and the corresponding actions necessary to accomplish them.

- By when do you want to achieve this goal?

- What obstacles can be expected?

- What are the solutions to the obstacles?

# # 3    Let Go of Pain from Your Past

The third prerequisite to living a healthier lifestyle is letting go of all the failures, disappointments, hurts and blame of your past. Perhaps you failed to accomplish a particular goal or you experienced great disappointment due to the actions of someone significant in your life. Maybe something happened that was completely beyond your control or you trusted someone and they disrespected you; trampled on your emotions; crushed a portion of your heart; and a part of your self-esteem was scarred. Regardless of the situation(s) that may have caused you pain, you have to grieve it and leave it. The grieving process is vital to your ability to recover and move forward. Grieving will allow you to purge those negative emotions and free you from becoming critical and spiteful (malicious) during this process. Then forget about the blame game and only evaluate your part that contributed to the pain. Finally, you must let go and allow the wounds to heal. Prior circumstances in your life cannot be used as excuses for not moving on to a healthier standard of living. You cannot change what you or someone else said or did in the past. The only thing you can change is how you respond to the event or person from this moment forward. Forgive those that have hurt you and make a concerted effort to learn from their mistakes and yours. Then forgive yourself. Once you have forgiven that person and yourself, never focus your attention on or talk about the incident again. You have to close the door, lock it, and walk away forever. You must learn to walk in love with those who have hurt you. That's not easy. But it must be done for your own peace of mind because when you fail to forgive, you keep yourself in bondage to the person that caused the pain. Don't make that mistake. Life is too precious and you can't get back any of the time that you wasted in unforgiveness. I kept myself in bondage for many years. Today, I cannot find words that explain the liberation I felt when I let go of all that unforgiveness and heaviness. It was as though a weight had suddenly been lifted off of me and there had been an explosion of vigor and life forced into my veins. My lungs were uncontaminated and immediately I could breathe the crispness of fresh air – air that could only be inhaled in a place beyond understanding. The taste of liberation will never be forgotten. I wasted all of those years before I realized that in order to live a healthier lifestyle, I had to be released from bondages that restricted my ability to thrive in all areas of my life.

Emotional stress, in spite of its cause, can contribute to chronic health problems over time. Your body pays a huge physiological price for each minute that you feel anxious, tense, frustrated, and angry. When these feelings are first experienced, your body can respond appropriately. The problems develop when you are consistently going through these emotions because all health conditions, to some degree, are triggered by emotional stress. Therefore, it is important that you learn how to successfully control emotional stressors in your life and stop them from creating health conditions that are detrimental to your well-being. To help combat emotional stress, I discovered that it was necessary to breath deeply; exercise; spend time every day in meditation or doing relaxation techniques; practice visualization (see positive visions of yourself on a daily basis in the place you want or need to be); eat a well-balanced diet; and be truthful about your feelings – know yourself.

**The third prerequisite to living a healthier lifestyle is letting go of all the failures, disappointments, hurts and blame of your past.**

- What parts of this prerequisite do you need to incorporate in your life in order to live a healthier lifestyle? Who do you need to forgive and why?

- How will you achieve this goal?

- By when do you want to achieve this goal?

- What obstacles can be expected?

- What are the solutions to the obstacles?

## # 4   Be Genuinely Happy with Your Job and Accept Your Financial Status in Life

The fourth prerequisite to living a healthier lifestyle is that you must be genuinely happy with your job and able to accept your financial status in life.

In spite of your age or current job situation, if you are unhappy with the type of job you have it will have a direct impact on your physical, mental, and emotional health. Eventually, it will have a negative effect on all aspects of your life. When you are unhappy and irritable you are more prone to health conditions that frequently lead to ailments that cause you to have to take sick leave, which can contribute to additional tension and frustration. Then without realizing where you are headed, you will find yourself overtaken by negativity and disease. People with very low job satisfaction are more likely to develop depression and other mental illnesses.

If you find that your job is unfulfilling; not challenging anymore; or the work environment is not conducive for your mental health – changing jobs may be the solution. It certainly beats the anxiety you experience every day by going to a job that literally makes you sick. Therefore, take some time and reflect on what you really want to do with your life. After you have determined your career passion, develop a strategy for attaining it and put it into action.

When you are happy with your job, your attitude, demeanor and the quality of relationships in your life are good. Because you spend so much time at work, it is important that your job be something you value, want to do, and gives you a sense of purpose. Once your job satisfaction improves, your mindset will change and so will your overall health and wellness.

However, financial challenges can also have traumatic adverse effects on your relationships, lifestyle and health (whether or not you have achieved the pinnacle of your career or experienced a sudden reduction of income due to a job loss or retirement). In fact, depending on how the challenge is perceived and managed could make you stronger as a person or cause you tremendous psychological and physical distress. Therefore, regardless of where you are at this very moment financially, accept it and find innovative ways to live within it. That does not mean become complacent nor does it mean that you should try to compete with others that have things you desire to obtain. The green eye of envy and jealousy always leads to a slow painful death. Realize that you may not be where you want to be financially and there is nothing wrong with that. Keep working toward your goals but give up the stressful rat race of obtaining property, merchandise and services when you cannot afford them. Live within your earnings. Balance your checkbook and do not write checks or use debit cards when there is no money in the bank. Stay away from death by credit and borrowing money. Remember that you cannot borrow your way out of debt. (Using credit and borrowing money are only smart ways to utilize purchasing power when applied through the use of appropriate financial tactics.) When irrational financial decisions are made, the cost is cumbersome in terms of your mental capacities and your credit. Furthermore, the effects of such choices tend to seep into every other aspect of your life. Desiring to have nicer things is human. And you deserve such pleasures, but you don't deserve the additional stress and headaches associated with living above your income.

For that reason, develop creative strategies that will take you to the next economic level and stay focused as you achieve your objectives and maneuver through the plan. It will require time and a lot of hard work (another choice you will have to make). Just keep in mind that Rome was not built in a day but it did not take a lifetime either.

**The fourth prerequisite to living a healthier lifestyle is that you must be genuinely happy with your job and be able to accept your financial status in life.**

- What parts of this prerequisite do you need to incorporate in your life in order to live a healthier lifestyle?

- How will you achieve this goal?

- By when do you want to achieve this goal?

- What obstacles can be expected?

- What are the solutions to the obstacles?

# # 5   Remove Toxins from Your Body

The fifth prerequisite to living a healthier lifestyle is removing toxins (the root cause of many illnesses) from your body even though your body automatically detoxifies to preserve your well-being. Pollutants are everywhere (air, water, and food) and we cannot get away from them. Coupling toxins with skipping meals, poor eating habits, stress and depleting your body of the proper amount of water can have a negative impact on your health. In fact, feeling tired and drained of energy could be a side effect of toxins that have entered your body. Fatigue is one of the first tell-tell signs of overload. It can change your entire appearance from head to toe. And if truth be told, your face lacking that glow of radiance can be interpreted as an indicator that a problem may be emerging in your body. Therefore, if for no other reason than the one previously stated, at least every 6 months eliminate toxins from your body. According to my doctor, "This will improve your overall health and natural balance." After cleansing your system, you will feel healthier than you have in years and you may find that some of the aliments that you thought you had, no longer exist. But before detoxing, ask your doctor for personalize guidance in this area.

There are many ways to detox but the two techniques I use on a weekly basis are soaking in a jacuzzi (104°F) for twenty minutes and fasting. When in the jacuzzi, your body temperature elevates and produces perspiration which relieves your body of toxins through your pores. However, men I must caution you about frequently using the jacuzzi as a means of detoxing because immersing the testicles in extremely hot water can lower the sperm count and can contribute to fertility problems. On the other hand, if you are living on a budget, fasting is economically cost-efficient and has been associated with the healing process as well as longevity.

**The fifth prerequisite to living a healthier lifestyle is removing toxins (the root cause of many illnesses) from your body.**

- What parts of this prerequisite do you need to incorporate in your life in order to live a healthier lifestyle?

- How will you achieve this goal?

- By when do you want to achieve this goal?

- What obstacles can be expected?

- What are the solutions to the obstacles?

## # 6   The Ability to Love

The final and most essential perquisite for living a healthier lifestyle is having the ability to love. Everything you do for others and yourself must be motivated by love. And you must be so rooted and grounded in love to the point that you love and respect yourself enough to want to do what's right for your health. As stated earlier, no one else can make this decision for you. Sometimes, we find making sacrifices and loving others easier than sacrificing and displaying love towards ourselves. But there comes a time when you must realize that there are some things no one else in this life can do for you. Either you seize the moment and do it yourself or you miss the opportunity (many of which you will never be afforded to experience again). Making decisions about living a healthier lifestyle is embedded into every moment of your existence. You were given one body in this life and the choice is yours what to do with it. You can abuse it, neglect it, and shorten its lifecycle or you can love yourself enough to do everything within your power to preserve, maintain, and increase its longevity. The choice is yours. Healthy living requires an infinite series of choices.

From the beginning of time, man was told that the secret to longevity is:

- watch your tongue
- always tell the truth

- do what you know is right
- spend time doing good
- try to live in peace with everyone, and
- work hard at it

This antidote for longevity includes being given the ability to make choices in every area of your life and walking in love is the foundation that you must undergirt yourself with in order to do that. You can not just pretend that you love others or yourself. You must really love with genuine affection recognizing the following dynamics of love as you travel the path.

**Love is patient and kind.** Patience is a character trait that you must possess as you attack the challenges associated with becoming a healthier person. Your patience will be tested on more than one occasion (maybe several times a day). Pass the test. Life happens so don't take it so seriously. And during this process of change, you must display kindness to everyone, even when people speak negatively of you and tell you that, "You'll never change."

**Love is not jealous, boastful, proud or rude.** Since you have transformed your mindset (changed the way you think), jealousy, boastfulness, pride, and rudeness are a thing of your past. Those attributes are no longer a part of your temperament. You have realized that an attitude of patient endurance and humility is the key to achieving the goals you are striving toward. And it is your gentle quiet spirit within that will assist you in becoming a healthier person.

**Love does not demand its own way.** Having "your own way" is what has gotten you to the point that you are at right now. But you have taken the first and most important step which is admitting that something in your life must change. So you are taking on new thoughts, adding corresponding actions and will be doing things differently from the way you did them in the past. You are to be commended for making such a life altering decision.

**Love is not irritable and it keeps no record of when it has been wronged.** Because patient endurance has become a part of your new nature, things do not bother you the way they did in the past. And because of the gentle quiet spirit inside of you, you have forgiven those who have caused you pain. As a result, things don't get on your nerves or frustrate you as much anymore. You see life through a different set of lenses.

**Love is never glad about injustice but rejoices when the truth wins out.** You were wounded and heartbroken because of pain inflicted upon you. But when you found out that you had to forgive in order to free yourself of that bondage, you forgave and let go of the hold it had over your life. Now you rejoice with a glad heart.

**Love never gives up, never loses faith, is always hopeful and endures through every circumstance.** For years, you have tried to change but it did not work so you gave up. But this time, you have made up your mind that life as you have known it cannot remain the same. You accept the challenge and this time you are not giving up. You recognize that there is no quick fix. The changes you make must become a way of life. You will succeed in spite of what happens as you travel the road to becoming a healthier person. You believe in yourself and the decision you have made.

Each of us has been given the ability to do certain things well which includes becoming the person we were created to be.

**The final and most essential perquisite for living a healthier lifestyle is having the ability to love.**

- What parts of this prerequisite do you need to incorporate in your life in order to live a healthier lifestyle? What acts of love do you need to improve?

- How will you achieve this goal?

- By when do you want to achieve this goal?

- What obstacles can be expected?

- What are the solutions to the obstacles?

## Interesting Note

In earlier days, fruits, herb bearing seeds, fish, and bread were considered the main course of the meal. When was the last time you ate seeds as a part of your diet or as your main course? Did you know that even today, there are cultures such as the Navajo Indians, Hunzakuts, and Abkhazians that use seeds as a vital part of their diets and these cultures have never had a reported case of cancer when eating their traditional foods? Furthermore, the Hunzakuts reside in the Pakistan area and often live to celebrate their 100th birthday. In my opinion, that is remarkable. They must be doing something right in the areas of health preservation and food preparation.

I enjoy preparing food myself because I love to eat and as a result, I often search for unusual recipes. As a matter of fact, one day while on my quest for something different for dinner, I found an ancient bread recipe that required it be made of wheat, barley, beans, lentils, millet and spelt. Apparently, the consumers of this bread recipe lived during an earlier time in civilization and did not realize that this recipe contained B17, which in its purified form today, has been developed for cancer therapy. Blackberries, blueberries, grapes, strawberries, apples, peaches, and apricots also contain B17.

# 6:30AM

## LET THE DAY BEGIN

*As you read the following pages of this book about a typical day in the life of a person with a healthier lifestyle and the necessary corresponding actions, imagine yourself as the person being depicted between the pages. Draw upon patient endurance and humility as you become accustomed to a new way of living, not just existing.*

- Wake up at least an hour earlier than you need to get up to prepare for work – this means everyday (including Saturday and Sunday) at the same time. As you are lying in bed contemplating whether or not to hit the snooze button, pause for a moment and consider all the wonderful blessings in your life.

- Go to the bathroom. Wash your face with a mild face cleanser that responds well to your skin type, not soap. Many of the soaps on the market today contain detergent that is harsh and simply dries out the skin. I use a deep action cream cleanser that is oil-free and cleans deep down in the pores. It leaves a cool, refreshing tingle on my face. Then follow this up with a moisturizer that has a sun screen (SPF 30 if possible) as part of its ingredients.

- Brush your teeth for a minimum of 2 minutes with toothpaste that does not contain saccharin or red and blue dyes. We have all heard the news alerts about these substances causing cancer. Pleasant tasting natural toothpastes can be purchased in some grocery stores, pharmacies, and health food stores. They tend to cost more than your typical commercial brands but you are worth it. And have you ever read the warning labels on the back of the toothpaste tubes? This was brought to my attention by a person selling home products. Read the back of your toothpaste tube. You may be surprised to find out that toothpaste can be poisonous.

- Change your tooth brush every three months or sooner if bristles are worn out or bent; or if you get sick (with a fever); are coughing; have a throat infection; or gum infection etc.

- If you use a mouth wash, use a brand that does not contain alcohol. Some mouth washes contain 25% to 27% alcohol. That is more alcohol than in the average can of beer (3% to 5%). Mouth washes with high percentages of alcohol can actually cause you to have bad breath as well as contribute to the development of different kinds of cancer. Have you ever thought about why some mouth washes burn so bad? Or have you ever read the back of the bottle to see what other uses the product may have such as getting rid of dandruff. Are you serious? And we put this in our mouths?

- Drink at least 8 ounces of filtered water. I personally enjoy an 8oz cup of hot water on an empty stomach every morning. Your water doesn't have to be hot but it should be one cup of the three quarts of water the average person requires a day. To determine the amount of water you need per day, divide your body weight by 2. This is the amount of water in ounces you need per day. Now divide that number by 8. Eight ounces is considered one cup.

- And in case you are wondering whether or not you can count the number of cups of coffee or tea that you drink per day as a part of your water intake, the answer is, "No." They cannot be counted as a part of your daily water consumption.

- Coffee and tea have caffeine in them which increases the flow of urine from the body making it more difficult to remain adequately hydrated. Drink water.

- Purchase a water bottle from your local sporting goods shop that holds the daily recommended amount of water. These bottles are very economical, retail price about $4. Carry the bottle with you everywhere you go. My bottle goes from room to room when I am home, to work, on leisure trips, ball games, and shopping. Think about it. Your body is about 60% water. Your muscles and brain are about 75% each while your blood is 82% and your bones are about 25% water. Can you imagine what you are doing to yourself when you fail to supply your body with the recommended amounts of water each day? Can you image your arteries and brain clogging; your immune system not functioning properly; and the signs of aging? Drink water.

• The next step is exercising which is a vital part of a healthy lifestyle. However, before you start any exercise regiment, have a physical exam and talk to your doctor about the type of exercise best for you. To begin any exercise routine, always warm-up and stretch (even before walking).

• Regular exercise such as walking, running (jogging), aerobic fitness methods, biking (cycling), swimming, and dancing are not only beneficial for the cardiovascular system but also for building up and toning muscles, enhancing the elasticity of joints, and undoubtedly decreasing the likelihood of osteoporosis. Exercising can also cause new stem cells to grow in your brain.

• Walking is an excellent exercise. It is very stimulating. The duration of the walk (any exercise regime) should average 30 minutes at least three times a week. Then include some type of weight lifting in your program in order to tone your muscles. My typical routine consists of fast walking (4.3 mph) two miles on the treadmill everyday. Three times a week I include arm curls, leg extensions, and chest press. The results are invigorating. And people who walk receive wonderful benefits to their health such as major declines in diabetes and heart disease, reductions in high blood pressure, increases in bone density, stronger hearts, improvement in cognitive abilities, fewer signs of depression, lower possibilities of breast and colon cancer, and increases in physical performance. But don't just walk away at the end of your 30 minute routine, take a few minutes to allow your body to slowly cool down while stretching again.

• Running (jogging) increases your metabolism which assists the muscles and heart in functioning more efficiently. It can also help burn a large number of calories when losing weight. Generally, if running daily is part of your exercise routine, you find yourself consuming less food since you are exerting so much energy into the exercise itself. However, if your goal is to achieve weight loss, as stated earlier, the only way to successfully lose weight is to consume fewer calories than you burn, apart from the amount of exercise you do. The same degree of wellness can be attained by running on a treadmill or outdoors. As a matter of fact, a lot of distance-running athletes make use of the treadmill so as to save their legs from injuries that can occur when running on asphalt, rocks, and roadwork. However, there is a small discrepancy in calories burned between running on a treadmill or outdoors. When running outdoors, you will burn a few more calories than treadmill running (at the same speed) because of not having air resistance on the treadmill. In order for calories burned to be the same, set the treadmill at 1% elevation.

• Aerobic exercise is any movement that you can maintain longer than merely a few minutes as your heart, lungs, and muscles work overtime to become stronger. This type of exercising helps the flow of air in and out of the lungs. No other part of exercise science has been discussed as much as the benefits of aerobic exercise. Regular aerobic exercise will enhance your health, fitness, and cognitive function. It will help prevent cancer, osteoporosis, depression, diabetes, cardiovascular disease, and obesity.

• Biking is a great low impact exercise that allows you to burn lots of calories, strengthen your heart, tighten and tone your legs, hips, and build stamina. Fast and continual biking will give you an opportunity to burn as many as 750 to 1,000 calories per hour. Yet, the average person does not work that hard; therefore, burning 500 to 600 calories is a more realistic expectation. Nevertheless, the amount of calories you burn will fluctuate significantly as determined by whether the bike you are riding is stationary or if you are riding a bike outdoors; how much energy you are exerting; and the efficiency of the bike.

• Swimming is an exercise that also burn lots of calories. It is easy on the joints and enhances cardiovascular health as it lowers your body temperature and rejuvenates you. This exercise can be continued safely into your senior years. It requires no ground impact; therefore, your joints are saved from injury. In fact, the Arthritis Foundation clearly advocate swimming and water exercises because of there being no ground impact involved in the exercise, so much so that they serve as patrons for water classes in various areas across the United States. Water aerobic classes are also desirable because swimming is an exercise that builds endurance and muscle mass. And it is one of many exercises that the entire family can enjoy together. When swimming you can burn from 500 to 650 calories per hour depending on how well you swim. And, as a matter of fact, you tend to burn more calories from just playing around in the water.

- Dance is an extraordinary kind of exercise which offers the heart-healthy advantages of aerobics as you participate in a more social kind of activity. It has become very popular in many gyms and dance studios. Putting exercise to music is a fantastic notion because it seems like an effortless cardio workout but it is so important because dancing can assist in the development of bone density and reducing the risk of osteoporosis. When dancing and enjoying yourself, endorphins will be released in your body and reduce your blood pressure. Dance is a wonderful anti-aging exercise.

- Ballroom dancing is considered one of the most elite styles of dance. It appears romantic and graceful but it is not easy. It is a heart pumping workout that improves your posture, sense of balance, and flexibility. Some of the dances included in this category are the Tango, Waltz, Foxtrot, Viennese Waltz, Quickstep, Cha-Cha-Cha, Rumba, Samba, and Jive.

- Belly dancing involves quick, rolling movements of the hips and abdomen. It strengthens the back and the muscles of the pelvic floor. Dance moves tend to start out moderate but can become faster and more aerobic as time progresses. This is an excellent exercise for fighting abdominal flab (when your age is forty something and older) and gently increasing core strength.

• Line dancing is regarded as a low impact dance yet it certainly has the ability to increase your heart rate. Music from various genres such as R&B, Latin, jazz, swing, or urban nightclub can be used when line dancing. Dances that can be performed in a line include the Waltz, Fox trot, Swing, Jive and Boogie, with and without partners.

• Latin dance with its fast pace is popular on the floor in nightclubs and health clubs as well. The dances are more sensual with a lot of sexy hip movement and rhythmic expression.

• Others types of dance that you may find appealing are ballet, jazz, tap, hip-hop, modern, swing, break dance, step, and folk.

• Exercising decreases the chances of having osteoporosis, yet, this condition has been diagnosed in millions of Americans. Today, 80% of women and 20% of men are osteoporosis sufferers.

• Osteoporosis is a disease that occurs when bones become more and more fragile and can be expected to break due to calcium loss and a decline in density. People with osteoporosis have no warning signs except weakening of the bones. As a result, a person can have this medical condition and not be aware of it. Osteoporosis can have an effect on any bone in the body. However, the greatest concerns are associated with possible fractures of the hip and spine. An astounding 1.5 million bone fractures a year are caused by osteoporosis which includes more than 300,000 fractures of the hip. Osteoporosis can necessitate surgical treatment and hospitalization. It can also lead to loss of height and spinal abnormality.

• Smoking and excessive alcohol or drug use can become contributing factors to the formation of osteoporosis. A lot of drugs impede the body's capacity to store and synthesize calcium.

• Eating a balanced diet rich in calcium and vitamin D helps to prevent osteoporosis. And weight-bearing exercises not only strengthen muscles, but also contribute to an increase in bone density. Having a higher bone density assists with decreasing the effects of osteoporosis.

• Drink at least another 8 ounce glass of water to replace water that your body used during exercise. Try to avoid drinking hot tap water due to metals in your pipe getting into the water. Drink filtered water instead. I use reverse-osmosis filters with activated carbon filtration for drinking water.

• Now it's time to hit the shower where you have installed a shower filter that eliminates chlorine from the water. When filters are not used, chlorine can enter your body through the steam you inhale and the pores of your skin. It is a very harsh chemical that can dry out your hair and skin. By installing filters, you are decreasing the possibility of exposure and absorption of chlorine in your body. Chlorine has been associated with heart disease and different types of cancer. I use a GE shower filter that also reduces the unpleasant smell of chlorine, rust, and other sediments.

• When thinking in terms of damaged hair, temporary, semi-permanent, demi-permanent, permanent coloring, lighteners, and bleaches have chemicals that can do away with and/or cover up pigments naturally found inside the hair shaft. Use of hair dyes can result in a range of adverse effects including temporary skin irritation and allergy, hair breakage, skin discoloration and unexpected hair color. Lead poisoning may also be a more serious health consequence of hair color usage. I used blonde hair coloring for several years. And when I completed a tissue mineral analysis, the amount of lead found in my body was off the chart. Needless to say, that is not a practice that I continue today.

• Use an unscented, detergent-free moisturizing body wash instead of soap as you shower.

• Men exfoliate your face two or three times a week prior to shaving unless the directions on the exfoliating scrub state otherwise. You will observe an enormous difference in the feel of your skin.

• Ladies, I recommend that you wait until you are ready to remove your makeup at night before you exfoliate.

• Brush your teeth again with natural tooth paste. Rinse.

- The water filter you have installed may also help eliminate fluoride from the water. I am sure you have heard of many areas in the country adding fluoride to the water supply in order to strengthen teeth and protect against cavities. These water supplies are being fluoridated on the assumption that all people, regardless of their body weight, age or state of health, require the same fluoride level. The debate about this belief is widespread and what is not being discussed is that the build up of large amounts of fluoride in the body can be hazardous to your health. The accumulation of fluoride in the body can come from many sources such as industrial air emissions, foods grown, manufactured or cooked in fluoridated areas, fluoridated water, toothpaste, fluoride tablets, mouthwash, tea, and Teflon cooking utensils. This build up of fluoride in the body can cause aches and stiffness in muscles and bones. It may also affect vitamins being taken and contribute to headaches, fatigue and some digestive problems such as irritable bowel syndrome.

- Eat a piece of fresh fruit as you are getting dressed since fruit should be eaten alone for better digestion. I love eating a fresh apple or pear before breakfast.

- Fruit breaks down very rapidly and when it is eaten too quickly following other foods, it will be stopped in the digestive tract and ferment.

- Get dressed. Wear garments that not only flatter your figure (body type) but also the shade of your skin. Now you may be wondering, what does your appearance have to do with living a healthier lifestyle? The answer is everything. Your physical appearance has a tremendous effect on your mindset, what you think about yourself.

• Women, put on your makeup before you leave the bathroom. Whether or not to wear makeup is not an option. The days of plain, bare foot, and pregnant are a thing of the past. You want to look your best every waking moment and makeup can give you that added edge that accents your beautiful skin. Consider it a part of your attire. It is just as vital as wearing under garments. Its importance can be viewed like that of MasterCard, "Don't leave home without it." Use a liquid-based foundation with shimmer or a cream blush or bronzer instead of mineral powders. Particles from powders can be inhaled and get into your lungs. And for your lips, forget about the lip gloss. Apparently, petroleum jelly is what gives lip gloss its shine and petroleum jelly is a derivative of oil drilling. But here is the kicker: When applied to your lips, you end up eating it, which is basically the same as drinking gasoline. The use of many petroleum jelly products has been banned in Europe due to the concern that it may be linked to cancer. Instead, use a lipstick that has a moisturizer and vitamin A.

• Men please do not drown in the bottle of cologne because the smell will intensify over time. Apply a small amount of cologne on your torso and one drop behind each ear. By doing this, when a woman invades your space to talk to you, she will definitely take note of your scent because it will radiate from those areas.

- Shoes should be clean with no chipped or worn-down heels, should I continue? You know how to look good. Select carefully the fashion styles you choose to wear. But remember that every style should not be worn by all people. And don't get lost in a time zone. As my Uncle Joe use to say, "Just because you're getting older doesn't mean you have to look old." (Uncle Joe was sixty years old with the look and vitality of a person in their mid-forties when he made the previous statement.) The interesting part of all of this is that Uncle Joe was right.

- Allow me to elaborate a step further on this notion and state that if you have not updated your hairstyle, wardrobe or shoes in three years or more, the time has come for you to get a makeover. Arrange a date at your local hair salon and do something extraordinary with your hair. Color (lighter is better) and a cut always bring the word "chic" into your appearance. Then sit back and allow your stylist to be creative. However, take your own makeup with you because most counter samples in department stores and salons are contaminated with everything from strep bacteria to E Coli. Next, shop until you drop and remember that buying new clothes does not have to be expensive. Make purchases during seasonal sales but buy items that can be worn all year (especially if you have to stick to a budget). Opt for pieces that you would not typically buy or come across in your wardrobe. Then get dressed, look in the mirror and tell yourself how attractive you are. This makeover should cause you to feel more gorgeous (handsome) and thrilled about your new look. After all, the first impression (yours) is the most important one.

**What practices from the 6:30 AM hour do you need to incorporate in your morning routine in order to live a healthier lifestyle?**

- How will you achieve this goal?

- By when do you want to achieve this goal?

- What obstacles can be expected?

- What are the solutions to the obstacles?

## 8:00 AM

**NOTE:** *No food in and of itself is wrong to eat. It is how the food is prepared; the amount of consumption; and whether or not you should be consuming the food item that causes the difficulty.*

- It's time to prepare breakfast. Avoid cooking with hot tap water and make healthy food selections.

- Eating a bowl of soup is a great way to jumpstart your day. Not only are you putting something hot in your stomach but you are reducing your intake of calories. Many chicken broth based soups have less than 100 calories. Just be careful about the sodium content. I make my soup from scratch in order to control the amount of each ingredient. Soups are very fulfilling and great appetizers. Having a bowl of soup as your first course will probably reduce the amount you consume during breakfast. Try eating at least one bowl of chicken broth based soup a day and observe the difference in your weight. You will be pleasantly surprised.

- Limit the number of eggs you consume due to the cholesterol intake. One raw egg contains about 213 mg of cholesterol. For that reason, try to eat no more than 3 organic eggs per week. When I prepare scramble eggs, I use one raw egg and the appropriate amount of egg whites that equal a second egg. Specific measurements can be found on the carton. That gives me the equivalent of two eggs but I am not getting the additional cholesterol.

- Blueberry or apple pastries, glazed donuts and chocolate chip pecan cookies; how can something taste so good to you yet be so bad for you? The problem is too much sugar and yeast. In fact, yeast feeds on sugar from the foods we eat and can cause abdominal bloating. Women, you know what I am talking about. If you are like most women, bloating can add those additional inches in the belly area making you look as though you are pregnant. And no one in their right mind desires to look pregnant when they are not.

- Stop and think for a moment about the number of foods that actually contain yeast. The list is extensive; therefore, control your consumption. Too much yeast could also release toxins in your blood and cause you to experience confusion, irritability, and low energy levels.

- You also need to monitor the amount of sugar you are eating. As a result, foods such as white bread, potatoes, popcorn (my favorite), pasta, corn, and cereals must be accounted for since they convert into sugar.

- White bread absorbs quickly and produces a rise in blood sugar more rapidly than whole grain bread. In addition, difficult movement of the bowels is a side effect associated with the texture of white bread when digestion is taking place. The 100% whole grain bread is definitely a better choice.

- Canned fruits have a huge quantity of sugar as well. Strive to develop a routine of eating only fresh fruits.

- Canned foods and aluminum. Our bodies can handle low levels of aluminum; however, we must ensure that the levels remain low. Therefore, do not use aluminum foil to cook or store foods and limit your consumption of canned food products due to the risk of aluminum toxicity. Foods (especially acidic foods like tomatoes and citric fruits) stored or cooked in aluminum cans or pots can contain up to 4mg of aluminum per serving.

- Aluminum toxicity can affect the nervous system displaying itself in symptoms such as inability to sleep, nervousness, emotional instability, memory loss, and headaches.

- Digestive problems, muscle aches, speech problems and anemia may be the result of aluminum toxicity.

- Antiperspirants and stainless steel cookware are sources of aluminum, as well as, hemorrhoid and diarrhea medications and buffered aspirin. Salts found in cake mixes, frozen dough, pancake mix, and self-rising flour also have aluminum in the ingredients.

- Processed cheese and beer (in aluminum cans) contain aluminum as well. One individually wrapped slice of cheese can contain up to 50 mg of aluminum.

- There are tests that you can have to help you monitor nutritional and toxic elements in your body. I had a hair analysis completed and the findings were breathtaking.

- The better cookware to use is cast iron because it adds iron to your food as it cooks; however, glass (without non-stick surfaces) and enamelware are also good choices, none of which react chemically to foods.

- Cookware with non-stick coated surfaces can release toxins into your food when heated above certain temperatures.

- Select beverages such as water, homemade lemonade, and unsweetened green tea as substitutes for soft drinks or other drinks that have a lot of extra sugar in the form of high-fructose corn syrup.

- Sports drinks, fruit drinks, and soft drinks (soda or pop) are loaded with sugar. In helping my son complete a research project on different types of drinks, we discovered that some soft drinks have as much as three tablespoons of sugar in them. For that reason, it is vital that your calorie intake be well thought-out when drinking beverages.

- Drinking coffee or black tea is another story. Consuming either of the two beverages with meals can cause the stomach to empty into the small intestine before stomach acids have properly broken down foods. When this occurs, indigestion is usually the result.

- Remember, for every cup of coffee or black tea that you consume, drink an equal amount of water in order to minimize its effect on your body.

- A typical American's intake of sugar is about 150 pounds per year. Eating habits tend to be so centered-around sugar that diseases such as heart disease, kidney stones, osteoporosis, and obesity are more prevalent today than ever. Consumption of this magnitude is especially disturbing because the immune system can become weakened and unable to fight against viruses.

- Obesity is occurring in astronomical proportions in the United States. The frequency of obesity in children is noticeably greater than before with about 20% of children identified as overweight or obese; 1 out of 3 children are overweight while 1 out of 5 have been identified as obese. The numbers are staggering.

- Obese children are at greater risk for heart disease, cancer, lung disease and diabetes. In fact, the life expectancy of obese children may be below that of their parents.

- A new presidential proposal devised to reverse child obesity is a major initiative underway. The report from the White House Task Force on Childhood Obesity clearly states an objective to decrease childhood obesity by 15%. To achieve this, the proposal presents seventy suggestions for early childhood, parents and caregivers, school meals and nutrition education, for an entitlement to utilize healthy food and for boosting physical activity.

- The effects of obesity are becoming evident in other areas of life as well. The United States armed forces currently advise that 1 out of 4 Americans aged 17 to 24 is "too heavy" to join the military service.

- The White House also has a proposal to turn around this phenomenon with a very specific objective of which the Center for Disease Control will report child obesity rates every two years.

- The average amount of body fat (articulated as percentage of body fat) is between 25% to 30% in women and 18% to 23% in men. Women with over 30% body fat and men with over 25% body fat are regarded as obese.

- Body mass index (BMI) is a measure of body fat based on height and weight that applies to both adult men and women. There are several websites on the internet where you can calculate your body mass index. You simply enter your height and weight and click compute BMI. Having a BMI of 30 or above is considered obese.

- Diabetes is a disease that has affected over eighteen million people in the United States. Thirteen million people have been diagnosed;

whereas another five million people have diabetes that has not been detected. A diagnosis of diabetes is made every year for over one million people age twenty or older. Diabetes is not contagious.

• Diabetes is a disease associated with your metabolism; how your body uses digested food for development and energy. A large amount of the food we consume is broken down into glucose, a form of sugar in the blood. Glucose is the chief source of energy for the body. It goes into the bloodstream after digestion where it is used by cells.

• Type 1 diabetes is an autoimmune disease. An autoimmune disease is the outcome when the body's system to combat infection (the immune system) goes against a part of the body. In Type 1 diabetes, insulin-producing beta cells in the pancreas are destroyed by an attack of the immune system. As a result, the pancreas will produce a small amount or no insulin. When a person is diagnosed with Type 1 diabetes, insulin must be taken on a daily basis in order to live. Type 1 diabetes occurs just as often among males and females; however, it is more widespread in whites than in nonwhites.

• Type 2 diabetes is diagnosed most often in 90% of people with diabetes. It has been linked to growing older; being overweight (more than 80% of people with diabetes are overweight); a family history of diabetes; prior gestational diabetes history; lack of physical activity; and ethnicity. And if truth be told, more and more children and adolescents are being diagnosed with Type 2 diabetes.

- A third type of diabetes is Gestational diabetes. It occurs during pregnancy. Once a female has gestational diabetes, there is a 20% to 50% chance that she will develop Type 2 diabetes within the next five to ten years. Similar to Type 2 diabetes, Blacks, American Indians, Hispanic Americans, and females with a family history of diabetes are more likely to be diagnosed. The highest percentage of diabetes in the world is found among American Indians.

- Always eat a good breakfast. Protein (chicken, turkey, fish) should be eaten first, if you have any, for better absorption. Your stomach must work a lot harder to break down proteins (especially red meat) than other foods. And try to limit yourself to one protein meal a day. Eat red meat sparingly. Which meal you include protein in is your choice.

- Eating too much processed meat raises the risk of pancreatic cancer, states new research conducted at the University of Hawaii. They followed 200,000 men and women for seven years and found that individuals who consumed the most processed meats (hot dogs and sausage) displayed a 67% increased risk of pancreatic cancer over those who ate little or no meat products. **AVOID EATING PROCESSED MEATS** such as hotdogs, sausage, deli meats, bologna, salami, lunch meats, bacon, beef jerky, pastrami, etc. These products contain sodium nitrate which is known as a cancer causing agent.

- Remember to chew every bite at least 20 times. Take time to savor the food; taste it; and enjoy the experience of the various consistencies and textures that each food brings to your senses. Don't rush through your meal.

- Should you choose to have water or a beverage with your meal, drink something hot or at room temperature; no more than 8 ounces. Again, this will assist the digestive process.

- The way your stomach works when you are eating can be compared to you baking a cake in the oven. The oven must heat to a certain temperature before putting the cake batter in it. (Your stomach becomes a certain temperature as you eat a meal.) Let's assume that you have changed your mind and no longer desire to bake a cake, so you turn the oven off. Now the oven begins to cool down. (Your stomach cools down as you drink cold beverages during your meal.) A few minutes later, you get a telephone call from your significant other who is bringing a guest home for dinner and you are asked to prepare a chocolate cake of which you always receive numerous compliments – you turn the oven on again in order for it to reheat to the appropriate temperature that is needed for baking a cake. (Your stomach must reheat when you start eating again. The heating process will continue until it reaches the exact temperature needed to assist in the digestive process again. This cycle repeats itself every time you eat and drink – heat up, cool down, reheat, cool down, reheat, etc.).

- If your breakfast includes hitting a fast-food restaurant on the way to work, plan to make careful selections. Here are a few healthier choices: Dunkin Donuts' Blueberry Bagel; McDonald's Egg McMuffin; Burger King's Ham Omelet Sandwich; Jack in the Box's Breakfast Jack; and Starbuck's Low Fat Bran Muffins.

- Try to stay away from croissants, biscuits, bacon, sausage, hash browns and cheese because they will pack on calories, fat and cholesterol. Drink water, unsweetened green tea, or coffee. The debate about whether or not to drink coffee is very controversial, so if you are going to drink it, do it in moderation. Then have a glass of water afterwards because coffee is a diuretic.

- Vitamins and supplements should be included in your daily routine. But with all the hype about which vitamins and supplements are better for you, what should you do? Taking a daily multivitamin, an extra vitamin D supplement, and Omega 3 supplement is a great way to ensure that you are getting the nutrients you need to be healthy but consult your physician before adding supplements to your diet.

- Prepare a filtered water bottle to take with you to work. Make sure that your water bottle is clean. This will keep your water fresh. If you drink directly from your bottle, you may need to do some additional cleaning at night and allow it to air dry before refilling it the next morning.

**What practices from the 8:00 AM hour do you need to incorporate in your morning routine in order to live a healthier lifestyle?**

- How will you achieve this goal?

- By when do you want to achieve this goal?

- What obstacles can be expected?

- What are the solutions to the obstacles?

## 8:30 AM

- As you are driving to work, think about good things. Many people use this as a time to listen to motivating words or songs. Your preference may be classical music or jazz. If you are the type of person that must hear the news report first thing in the morning, immediately after you receive your update, redirect your attention to motivating words or mellow music in your vehicle. The idea is to remain calm and think about things that are pleasant. Organize your thoughts about the activities you will embark upon during the day; how you will approach people; and how you will accomplish the many tasks that are waiting.

- There are several activities that you should avoid while driving because they are distracting and could cause serious accidents.

- The first thing to avoid is eating difficult to manage foods. Have you ever seen people trying to put condiments on sandwiches while driving down the road? They use one hand and their mouth to rip open the condiment. Then they squeeze out the condiment and try to evenly spread it on the bread as the rest of the sandwich is falling apart in their lap. The next task is picking up the sandwich as they replace the paper wrap around it so there will be no spills on their clothes. They are constantly not focusing on their driving during this process. The better thing to have done would have been to pull into a parking space after receiving their order; put the condiments on the sandwich; eat the sandwich; then resume driving. On the other hand, there are people that eat an entire meal from a To-Go plate using a fork. They not only eat while waiting at red traffic lights but also as they are driving. They look down, taking their eyes off the road every time they scoop up another fork of food. And don't let the food begin to fall off the fork, they lean towards the steering wheel and try to catch it with their mouth. This is a very dangerous situation.

- Ladies please avoid putting on makeup while driving. As you recall, makeup should be applied before you leave the bathroom. We've all seen the female looking in her rearview mirror putting on mascara but to be applying eyeliner is absolutely absurd. Consider how skillful one must be to keep eyeliner straight and the number of seconds the focus must be on the eye of which the liner is being applied. If it is one of those mornings and you are running late, wait until you get to the office and park the car. Then apply your makeup. If you are already late a couple more minutes won't make that big of a difference.

- The same safety measures discussed about makeup also apply to brushing your hair and shaving. It takes only a few minutes to accomplish each task. Do not jeopardize your safety or the safety of others by taking care of personal grooming while driving. Brush your hair or shave before you start your car or wait until after you have parked your vehicle.

- Flossing the teeth – who would have ever thought that someone would actually try to floss their teeth as they were driving? It happens and the person is using his (her) elbow and/or knees to steady the steering wheel. No where in the driver's manual does it stipulate that any body part other than the hands may be used to manipulate the steering device. Oral hygiene is important but it does not warrant behavior similar to a circus act while operating your car. Think safety first.

- Changing clothes is also something that you really should avoid when driving. Remove jackets and sweaters before getting into the vehicle to prevent getting overheated. But how many times have you seen males changing clothes in the car as they drive? I assumed they had just finish working out or completing some school athletic activity. Yet, what I couldn't figure out is why they did not put on the other set of clothing before they got into the car. I actually observed one guy putting on a t-shirt as he drove next to me on the interstate. For a few seconds, his entire face was covered. Those few seconds could have made the difference between life and death in an accident. And it doesn't stop there. I have seen young guys that wear two and three pairs of shorts underneath their long pants taking the pants off while waiting at the traffic light. Why is that necessary? Wait until you are in a more appropriate environment to change clothes.

- Cell phones. There have been many occasions when I have gone around cars on the interstate and in local traffic where the driver is weaving across the line or not traveling at least speed limit to find that they are holding the cell phone in one hand as they gesture with the other hand (leaving the steering wheel unattended) or texting. A better choice for cell phone usage is the hands-free devices. As far as sending text messages while driving, it is against the law in most states. **DO NOT TEXT AND DRIVE.**

- Everyday we must multi-task in order to keep up with the fast pace of our work environments. It has become so second nature that unfortunately we find ourselves multi-tasking even when we are driving. This does not legitimize it by any means; it is a very dangerous practice. When we eat, drink, talk on the cell phone and drive at the same time, how much focus are we really putting towards braking, reaction time, and following distance? Multi-tasking is not a practice that should be utilized when operating a vehicle.

- Reading books or reports while driving is another disaster waiting to happen. How many times have you seen people reading as they drive down the road? Even if they are reviewing information for an important meeting that they are going to, they are splitting their focus in two different directions. And the document review will be absolutely pointless if they have an automobile accident and never make it to the meeting. What about the person who reads a novel while waiting at red traffic lights? I have been behind drivers that were so engaged in the books they were reading that when the traffic light turned green for traffic to move forward, they just sat there – reading their book. Of course they have a reality check when drivers of other vehicles start sounding their horns but it should never get to that point. Drivers can receive careless driving tickets for reading and driving.

**What practices from the 8:30 AM hour do you need to incorporate in your morning routine in order to live a healthier lifestyle?**

- How will you achieve this goal?

- By when do you want to achieve this goal?

- What obstacles can be expected?

- What are the solutions to the obstacles?

## 8:45 AM

- Speak to people and smile at them when you arrive at work. The first few minutes you spend with co-workers each day has a vast effect on the morale of the workplace. In addition, your body language telegraphs every thing about your mood. Start the day right. Smile. Walk around your workplace tall and confident. Let people observe that today is going to be a great day and it begins with you.

- Work to the best of your ability. Be a good worker, a person that does not need to be ashamed.

- Guard your mouth if you think you may be tempted to indulge in conversation that is counter productive or hurtful in any way.

- Place the water bottle on your desk and take a drink every time you look at it.

- In order to increase my productivity during the day, I write a "To Do" list of things that need to be accomplished.

- Then I prioritize and organize each item on the list from most important or current deadlines to items with less significance that should be accomplished. Similar items are categorized together.

- Next monitor interruptions such as unannounced visitors and unscheduled phone calls. If your office is like mine, people are always dropping by just to chat. This waste a lot of valuable time that could be used to complete important tasks. In order to monitor disruptions when people come into my office, I set the alarm on my cell phone to go off every ten minutes. I pull my list back out and review the items on it. Then I refocus and get back to the task at hand. Another way to handle constant disruptions is to continue working without giving eye contact as the person makes conversation in your office. Usually within a couple of minutes after seeing that he (she) does not have your undivided attention, he (she) will leave. Keep in mind that most disruptions are not emergencies.

- Another good rule of thumb is to always verify appointments by a phone call prior to leaving the office. By calling first, you make sure the business meeting is still on and that parties involved will be arriving at the scheduled time. If there is going to be a delay, you may have time to complete another task on your list before leaving the office.

- Every time you finish a task, mark it off the list. By doing this you can see exactly how much you are accomplishing and what is left to complete.

- At the end of the day, revisit the "To Do" list in order to determine how many items have not been completed and what new tasks you added to the list during the day.

- Write those items on tomorrow's list. If several items were not completed and you worked meticulously all day, obviously you had more tasks to complete than could be accomplished in an eight hour work day.

- Adjust the number of items on the list that will be accomplished tomorrow taking into account that there are twenty-four hours in a day; at least eight of those hours are typically spent at work while the other sixteen hours are your time that should not be infringed upon by completing tasks that are on the "To Do" list.

**What practices from the 8:45 AM hour do you need to incorporate in your morning routine in order to live a healthier lifestyle?**

- How will you achieve this goal?

- By when do you want to achieve this goal?

- What obstacles can be expected?

- What are the solutions to the obstacles?

## 10:00 AM

- Eat a mid-morning snack. If you have a desk at work, you may have a snack drawer. Keep snacks on hand that provide nutrients. Try to make sure that some snacks contain protein as well as carbohydrates to better sustain your blood sugar level and curve your appetite until lunch. However, eat only one kind of fruit at a time, as much as you want. If you desire to eat a different kind of fruit, wait one hour for better digestion. Apples and peanut butter; yogurt and fruit; and vegetables make wonderful snacks.

- Keep in mind, fruit should not be eaten less than an hour before lunch because it really has a way of suppressing your hunger.

- When thinking in terms of food combining and digestion, melons (and I love watermelons) are best eaten alone because they combine with no other food (melons tend to break down faster than other foods). I have found this to be an excellent practice. In fact, I have also found that for better digestion, it's best not to combine different types of melons.

- Even though you have been drinking water periodically all morning, make sure you drink another 8 ounces before you eat lunch. It can decrease your appetite.

- Tea, coffee, and lemonade should never be used as substitutes for water simply because they are made with water.

**What practices from the 10:00 AM hour do you need to incorporate in your morning routine in order to live a healthier lifestyle?**

- How will you achieve this goal?

- By when do you want to achieve this goal?

- What obstacles can be expected?

- What are the solutions to the obstacles?

## 12:00PM

- Lunch should be your largest meal of the day.

- Eat a bowl of soup with a chicken broth base to curve your appetite.

- During your main course, eat protein (chicken, turkey, or fish) first, if you have any. Remember to chew every bite at least 20 times. Don't rush through your meal.

- Drink a beverage at room temperature (no more than 8 ounces).

- Food combining should be considered. It is **NOT** recommended that high starch foods such as potatoes, yams, lima beans, corn, pasta, squash, and brown rice be combined with protein. A better combination is high starches with low starches (i.e. greens, peppers, bean sprouts, cucumbers, brussel sprouts, broccoli, mushrooms, cabbage, lettuce, cauliflower and string beans); and a third combination would be low starches with proteins.

- If you take your lunch to work in a plastic container make sure that the container does not have the numbers "3" or "7" in a triangle on the bottom. Containers with this marking have Bisphenol (BPA), a toxic chemical used in some plastics. When heated in a microwave, the chemical is released into the food. BPA has been linked to cancer and certain harmful effects on the brain.

• Instead, pack lunches in plastic containers that do not contain BPA, glass or plastic lunch bags.

• Heating food in microwaves should be limited to glass containers.

• If lunch consist of a trip to a fast-food restaurant choose grilled, broiled or steamed foods over fried. Order regular or junior meals instead of "biggie" meals and substitute a baked potato (minus the cheese, sour cream, butter, and bacon) for french fries. Sub sandwiches, pitas, wraps, and burritos are also excellent choices if you do not include mayonnaise and cheese. Special sauces, cheese, sour cream, butter, bacon, and mayonnaise have lots of calories, fat, and cholesterol.

• Include brain foods (complex carbohydrates) such as wild salmon (not farm raised), whole grain breads, avocados, tuna, Matcha (stone ground green tea), blueberries, strawberries, cranberries, apples, and spinach as part of your lunch menu. Brain foods boost memory; help you think clearly; and contribute to overall good health.

• Other brain foods include **WATER,** flaxseed oil, whole grain cereals, almonds, yogurt, blackberries, walnuts, raspberries, oatmeal, organic peanut butter, broccoli, red grapes, pumpkin seeds, cherries, dark chocolate, sardines, tomatoes, Acai berries, red cabbage, and eggplant.

- Eating complex carbohydrates is a great choice because it takes them longer to break down during the digestive process into simple sugars that our body can use. As a result, our bodies do not get a surge of energy and then energy levels drop. With complex carbohydrates, our bodies and brain receive a consistent amount of energy over time. Other complex carbohydrate foods include spaghetti, brown rice, root vegetables, whole grain cereals, yams, peas, and beans.

- If you have a large appetite, include a side salad (without bacon bits) with your meal. Order salad dressings on the side and remember that creamy dressings have more calories and fat in a single serving. Make salads the last portion of your meal to be eaten so that water in the lettuce does not dilute your digestive fluids. Besides, eating salads last will also curve your appetite for desserts.

- Drink no more than 8 ounces of water at room temperature or unsweetened green tea instead of soda.

- Spend the last thirty minutes of your lunch hour exercising your brain. There are numerous books and internet sites that have mind exercise puzzles such as crossword, lateral thinking, logic, brainteasers, sequence, word search, memory development techniques, recall tests, mental agility, observation, and mental reasoning tests. Completing these puzzles on a daily basis (repetition is the key) will stimulate and keep your brain active. Choose a variety of exercises in several categories in order to improve various mental faculties (attention, speech, memory, reasoning, sensory, and conscious choice) and different areas of the brain.

- After lunch, continue to drink your filtered water. Water is needed to keep your kidneys healthy. Kidney stones can form due to dehydration (a lack of water).

- A kidney stone is a solid piece of mineral material that develops inside the kidney or urinary tract out of substances in the urine. This typically occurs when there is a reduction in urine volume and/or additional stone forming materials in the urine. A tiny kidney stone may pass completely out of the body with little or no pain. However, some stones may cause blood to appear in the urine and a lot of acute pain in the abdominal or groin areas. Kidney stones affect 1 out of 20 people at various stages in the life cycle.

- When you become dehydrated from not drinking adequate amounts of water or by not sufficiently replenishing fluids in your body that you lost during vigorous exercises you increase the likelihood of the formation of kidney stones. These stones may also develop when the flow of urine has been obstructed. Additionally, urinary tract infections can contribute to the formation of kidney stones.

- Men are more likely to have kidney stones than females. The occurrence of kidney stones start to increase as men are in their 40s and the rate continues to rise until they are in their 70s. Once a person has more than one kidney stone, the probability of developing more stones is higher. And when a family history of kidney stones exist, the chances are greater for developing kidney stones. Caucasians are diagnosed with kidney stones more often than Blacks.

- When you think that you are hungry and it is not time for a meal, start with a glass of water before looking for a snack. You may find that what your body was really telling you was that it needed water. When the body feels depleted of water it may ask for food as a means of obtaining water since about 37% of our daily water intake is acquired from the foods we eat.

**What practices from the NOON hour do you need to incorporate in your daily routine in order to live a healthier lifestyle?**

- How will you achieve this goal?

- By when do you want to achieve this goal?

- What obstacles can be expected?

- What are the solutions to the obstacles?

## 3:00 PM

- Eat a mid-afternoon snack. Chocolate, chocolate, and more chocolate. Every afternoon, the more paperwork I found myself in at the office; the more I craved chocolate. I would actually search for a co-worker who I knew had chocolate candy bars if my desk drawer supply was empty. It was becoming a very bad habit and I attached guilt to it because I knew I should not be eating milk chocolate everyday. Then I discovered that chocolate has chromium in it which helps to stabilize blood sugar and increases energy. That's probably why I kept craving it. So I began my quest to find another snack that had chromium that I could substitute in the place of the chocolate. Eventually, I found it. Sunflower seeds were an easy substitute.

- You need to refuel your body, especially if your job is anything like mine and requires a great deal of stress or movement. Other healthy snacks include instant breakfast drinks; almonds (unsalted); trail mix; a hard-boiled egg; cereal bars; granola bars; popcorn (air-popped); pretzels; raisins; instant oatmeal; and soup cups (broth-based and low sodium).

- For a quick surge of energy, eat pineapples.

- Avoid snacks that provide empty calories such as cookies, crackers, candy, soda (pop), chips, french fries and other deep fried foods.

- Besides refueling your body, you also need to do stretching exercises at your desk to prevent back pain and increase your energy. Sitting at a computer for hours every day can cause serious medical problems. The way you sit, type, and hold the phone can damage your bones, joints, and muscles.

- Backaches and pains can be the end result of leaning forward over your desk for extended periods of time during the day. And just because you are not obese does not mean that you should become complacent about moving. There are a lot of skinny people that obtain osteoporotic fractures because they fail to exercise for strength and balance.

- To increase energy and prevent stiffness do stretching exercises. The following six exercises are included for your consideration.

- Stand up and sit down without using your hands. Repeat three times.

- Shrug your shoulders as you breathe deeply maintaining that position for five seconds. Release. Repeat three times.

- Lift both arms up shoulder height in front of you. Draw circles in the air with your hands as you count to ten. Next reverse the direction of the circles as you count to ten again. Shake out your hands.

- Release your upper body with a torso twist. Breathe in and as you blow out air, twist your body to the right and grab the back of your chair with your right hand, and grab the arm of the chair with your left. Gradually face forward. Repeat on the other side.

- As you are seated in your chair, stretch your legs out in front of you to complete five leg extensions. Make sure that your legs are parallel to the floor. You may have to hold the seat of your chair in order to support yourself. Next bend your feet and point your toes. Release. Repeat four more times.

- Look up to the ceiling to release tension in your upper body. This exercise can be completed by sitting in your chair or standing on your feet. Extend your arms over your head and interconnect your fingers. Rotate the palms of your hand upward as you raise your chin up, lean your head back, and look at the ceiling. Breathe in, exhale, and release.

**What practices from the 3:00 PM hour do you need to incorporate in your mid-afternoon routine in order to live a healthier lifestyle?**

- How will you achieve this goal?

- By when do you want to achieve this goal?

- What obstacles can be expected?

- What are the solutions to the obstacles?

## 5:00 PM

- During the drive home think about pleasant things. Don't bombard your thinking by listening to the news. You are already exhausted. Listen to music or something that will help you to unwind before you get home and face the challenges of being a parent; a spouse; or just life. Sing along with songs that are upbeat. The temperature in the car should be cool (even during the winter months) because warmer temperatures will make you want to sleep. If the sleep fairy does sprinkle dust in your eyes, have something available in the car to snack on such as nuts or an apple (something crunchy). You may have to roll the windows down and allow air to hit you in the face. But don't inhale exhaust fumes from the traffic more than a couple of minutes. Too much inhalation of diesel, lead and exhaust fumes (particles) is bad for your cardiovascular system. Should you have to stop and stretch your legs, drive to a gas station and get a bottle of cold green tea. The caffeine should give you a boost in energy. It is important that you think about your safety and the safety of others when you are operating a car. Too many accidents happen from people falling asleep while driving.

- With everything that you have going on in your life right now, hopefully, the sleep fairy sprinkling dust in your eyes is the only thing happening at this time and you are not one of millions of Americans suffering from sleep deprivation. Not sleeping enough or not sleeping well has high stakes attached to it. Your physical, mental and emotional health is at risk. Regardless of the cause, whether it is stressors of daily life, work, interpersonal relationships, or undiagnosed sleep disorders, sleep deprivation will rob you of more than the money in your wallet. On average, not being able to sleep for about 1 ½ hours at night will reduce your alertness (by more than 30%) the next day. It can also impair your memory as well as your ability to think and process information. So consider what may be happening to your body if your sleep has been interrupted every night for an extended period of time. The odds are stacking up against you.

- There is a higher mortality risk for people getting less than six to seven hours of sleep each night. In fact, when people get less than the recommended hours of sleep, their mortality risk is greater than the mortality risk of people who smoke, have high blood pressure, or heart disease.

- In addition, sleep loss may also be a contributing factor to obesity. That is why it is important to include getting plenty of rest (sleep) in any weight loss regime. Better sleep habits may contribute to you being able to achieve the goals of your weight loss plan.

- According to the American Sleep Disorder Association, there are more than eighty-five sleep disorders acknowledged in the United States. Those disorders affect more than seventy million people. Furthermore, about one-third of the American population suffers from insomnia but less than 10% have been diagnosed.

- And there is a huge scope of sleep disorders from snoring to sleep apnea. Chronic snoring has been linked to a higher rate of heart and brain-related illnesses. More than 45% of the population in the U.S. is included in this category. Of those, nearly half of them have sleep apnea.

- Over twenty million Americans (24% men and 9% women) have some degree of obstructed sleep apnea. Yet, only a small percentage of those have actually been identified and receive treatment.

- Sleep apnea is a warning sign for high blood pressure. It is unfortunate that many people with sleep apnea don't know they have it and have not been treated for sleep apnea or high blood pressure. If they would receive treatment it would greatly reduce their chances of having a stroke. Sleep deprivation is serious business.

- By now your water bottles should be almost empty.

**What practices from the 5:00 PM hour do you need to incorporate in your daily routine in order to live a healthier lifestyle?**

- How will you achieve this goal?

- By when do you want to achieve this goal?

- What obstacles can be expected?

- What are the solutions to the obstacles?

## 5:30 PM

- When you arrive at home, if your significant other is there, approach him (her) with caution. You don't know what he (she) has experienced today. Remember that a gentle touch, a smile and a right attitude will turn away anger. Caress, kiss, politely excuse yourself and keep moving. Change clothes and sit in your special place where you will not be disturbed for at least 20 minutes. This is not the time to read your mail. This is your down time to clear your mind – meditate. It is your time with the most important person in the world, yourself. Meditation is a type of mind-body therapy. People from cultures around the world have used it as a way of promoting healing. Today, some doctors recommend the use of meditation to lower blood pressure, reduce insomnia, breathe better and unwind from the daily pressures of life.

- Meditation is a harmless way to keep equilibrium between your physical, emotional and mental being. The benefits are tremendous. I always feel rejuvenated and busting with vitality afterwards. Others have reported feelings of happiness, improved learning ability or memory, emotional stability as well as a vast reduction in irritability, depression, mood swings and anxiety.

- The posture you take on during meditation is very important. Many physicians recommend a sitting position. However, my preference is lying down on my back in the middle of my bed in order to induce a relaxation response. You will need to decide the posture most appropriate for you (sitting, sitting cross-legged, semi-reclining, etc.).

- Making meditation a part of your daily routine will absolutely enhance your life. Choose a quiet place where you will not be disturbed by anyone. Turn off the cell phone and the telephone to eliminate their distractions. Then choose a focus word or phrase to repeat during the meditation process.

- The next step is easy. Close your eyes and concentrate. Block out all sounds and focus on your body. I loosen my muscles from feet to head one after the other by commanding each body part to relax. This process is repeated until tension from each body part is released. After letting go of any obvious tension, relax the rest of your body moving upward (feet, calves, thighs, buttocks, pelvic, stomach, lower back, middle back, upper back, chest, hands, arms, shoulders, neck, jaws, and eyes). Often the shoulders and the neck require a little more work or concentration. By this time, your breathing should be slow and you should be in a very flaccid state. Now repeat your focus word or phrase for the remainder of the 20 minutes. Meditation is a gentle process that restores us to our creator's realm of serenity.

- Finally the time has arrived for you to take an active part in the lives of others in your household, listen to the news, read the mail, etc.

- You want to continue drinking your water and ensure that you have 8-16 ounces prior to dinner.

**What practices from the 5:30 PM hour do you need to incorporate in your daily routine in order to live a healthier lifestyle?**

- How will you achieve this goal?

- By when do you want to achieve this goal?

- What obstacles can be expected?

- What are the solutions to the obstacles?

## 6:30 PM

- Try to eat dinner before 7:00 PM. After that time, eat a light salad or fruit.

- When cooking, follow cooking directions on back of packages for amount of time necessary to cook foods (especially vegetables) to make certain that food is not overcooked. You may be surprised how many foods you have overcooked and striped of nutrients. Overcooked foods lose over 60% of their nutrients and are harder to digest. I was reared with southern hospitality, soul food, and lot of overcooked meals. I can remember growing up around people cooking vegetables for at least an hour and now I realize that many vegetables require very little cooking time. When I started preparing foods using healthier methods, ingredients and cooking times, I was surprised at how different food taste. It was flavorful and appetizing.

- Eat a bowl of soup with a chicken broth base to curve your appetite.

- Then eat lean cuts of protein such as chicken, turkey breasts or fish, first. If you are a beef or pork eater (which I am not), limit your intake of red meat.

- A study on the effects of red meat was conducted by the American Cancer Society. One hundred fifty Americans were involved in the study over a period of ten years. This was the largest and most comprehensive study on red meat to date. Prolonged high consumption was described as an intake of at least three ounces daily for men and two ounces for women over a 10 year time period. One ounce would be equivalent to one fast food hamburger. The study cited one ounce per day for processed meat (one slice of bologna or four slices of bacon) five to six days a week for men and two or three times a week for women. The results of the study suggested that too much red meat will raise your risk of colorectal cancer.

- Another word of warning is related to seasoning your food. Do you sprinkle salt on your food before you taste it? A good rule of thumb is one teaspoon of salt per day. However, four to five teaspoons of salt is consumed by individuals every day and about seventy-three million Americans (one in three adults) have been diagnosed with high blood pressure. This includes about two million American teens and children and many are under-diagnosed.

- Eating salt **DOES NOT** cause high blood pressure. Our bodies need salt in order to help control our fluid balance and the way our muscles and nerves work. When we eat too much salt, our bodies eliminate it through our urine. However, in some people (especially the Black population, the elderly, and people with diabetes) eating too much salt will cause the blood pressure to rise because they are sensitive to salt. Many people are salt sensitive.

- High blood pressure can be the result of an underlying medical condition, stress, narrowing of the arteries or the body lacking necessary minerals such as potassium, magnesium or calcium.

- In 95% of people with high blood pressure the cause of the condition cannot be identified, while 5% of people with high blood pressure have been identified as having malfunctions in various organs such as the kidney, adrenal gland, or aortic artery. High blood pressure may run in some families and it occurs more often in the Black population.

- High blood pressure (referred to as HBP or hypertension) is defined as elevated pressure in the arteries. Your arteries carry blood from your heart to every other part of your body. Emotional stress is not high blood pressure; however, emotional stress can elevate your blood pressure for the moment while you are under great tension.

- When measuring your blood pressure, a normal reading is 120/80 or below. Pre-hypertension levels range from 120/80 to 139/89. On the other hand, your blood pressure is considered high if your numbers are 140/90 or greater. The top number represents the systolic blood pressure – the amount of pressure in the arteries when the heart contracts and forces blood onward into the arteries. The bottom number represents the diastolic pressure. This indicates the pressure in the arteries as the heart slows down after the contraction. If the systolic and/or diastolic blood pressure rises, you are at greater risk to develop heart disease, kidney disease, hardening of the arteries (atherosclerosis or arteriosclerosis), eye damage, and stroke (brain damage).

- When diagnosed with high blood pressure (hypertension), lifestyle adjustments in diet and exercise are important. Using too much salt, being overweight, failure to exercise, consuming too much alcohol or coffee, and smoking may negatively affect you. It is also important to comply with medication regimes. High blood pressure (hypertension) that is unattended or inadequately managed can impair blood vessels in the eye; thicken heart muscles and cause heart attacks, hardening of the arteries (arteriosclerosis), kidney failure, and strokes.

- High blood pressure (hypertension) is referred to as "the silent killer" because there may be no warning signs that anything is wrong for many years. Some people have no symptoms for decades. Then they find out that there is damage to certain vital organs as a result of high blood pressure.

- Please understand that you **DO NOT HAVE TO USE HAM HOCKS, SALT MEAT, FATBACK, BACON, CURED TURKEY LEGS, AND STREAK OF LEAN for flavoring in order for foods to taste good.**

- Instead of using table salt and the items just mentioned, I use a lot of salt-free herbs. The following is a list of herbs that really enhance the flavor of foods: Poultry: curry powder, basil, onion, garlic, oregano, paprika, parsley, poultry seasoning, thyme, rosemary, sage, and savory. Fish: bay leaf; basil, curry powder; garlic; onion, dill, thyme, paprika, parsley, and fennel. Vegetables: onion, parsley, pepper, basil, chives, dill, marjoram, thyme, and tarragon. For beans, rice, and pasta use basil, dry mustard, garlic powder, onion powder, black pepper, basil, thyme, and paprika. Ms. Dash Seasoning Blends are also salt-free.

- For butter, I use Butter Buds and Extra Virgin Olive Oil is added as a last ingredient to some dishes after cooking has been completed.

- Non-stick cooking sprays label themselves "fat free" but the labels are misleading. If you read the small print on the back of the can you say find a similar statement, "Adds a trivial amount of fat." The law permits a product that contains less than .05 grams of fat per serving to be labeled "fat free." However, in order for that to hold true, you could only spray for a third of a second in order to equal one serving. When coating cooking utensils, spraying about 5 seconds is normal which adds almost 7.5 grams of fat and 75 calories to your food. Therefore, mist cooking utensils sparingly.

- There is more monounsaturated fat than saturated fat in many non-stick cooking sprays. As a result, they are healthier choices than butter or margarine.

• Make your own non-stick cooking spray by combining organic vegetable oil and liquid lecithin. (A natural emulsifier, lecithin can be purchased at most health food stores.) Pour equal amounts of both ingredients in a spray bottle and shake well.

• Non-stick cooking oils are aerosols; sprays that contain propellants and solvents. Aerosols are inhalants and chronic exposure to inhalants can harm the brain, heart, lungs, liver, kidney and other parts of the nervous system.

• Heart Disease (Coronary Artery Disease). In order for the heart to function, the blood must provide oxygen and nutrients. The coronary arteries supply the heart's needs but are in danger of thinning as cholesterol deposits (plaques) increase within the artery. If the arteries thin a sufficient amount, the blood supply to the heart muscle may slow down. The slowing of blood flow to the heart will trigger pain (angina). When plaque ruptures, a person will have a heart attack which allows the formation of a blood clot. The clot will completely block the artery and stop blood flow to part of the heart muscle (that portion of muscle dies).

• Some of the risk factors linked to heart disease include: diabetes, family history, high blood pressure, smoking, high cholesterol, peripheral artery disease and obesity.

- Smoking is an addiction. Tobacco contains a very addictive drug called nicotine. As a result, it is not easy (although not impossible) to stop smoking. As a matter of fact, given the U.S. Surgeon General's report on the risk associated with smoking, millions of Americans have "kick the habit" and you must too, if you smoke, and intend to live a healthier lifestyle because roughly 440,000 deaths take place in the United States every year from smoking-related diseases; this accounts for nearly 1 out of every 5 deaths. The explanation rendered in regards to these deaths is that smoking significantly increases the possibility of developing lung cancer, heart attack, chronic lung disease, stroke, and other types of cancer. In addition, smoking may be the most unnecessary reason for breathing (respiratory) diseases within the United States.

- Cholesterol is an essential element for cell membranes and hormones such as estrogen and testosterone. The liver makes approximately 80% of the body's cholesterol. The other 20% is obtained from the foods we consume. We acquire a lot of cholesterol from our diets when we eat meat, poultry, fish, and dairy products. However, no cholesterol is obtained from eating foods derived from plants.

- LDL cholesterol has been identified as "bad" cholesterol, since high levels of LDL cholesterol are linked to a heightened probability of coronary heart disease. HDL cholesterol has been identified as "good cholesterol" because HDL cholesterol particles inhibit atherosclerosis. Total cholesterol levels are greatly influence by heredity and diet. Diets that contain a lot of saturated fats and cholesterol elevate the amount of LDL cholesterol in the blood. Saturated fats can be found in meat and dairy products. Make sure that you read the label on the back of bottle of vegetable oil because some are high in saturated fats.

- Ten million people in the United States are affected by peripheral artery disease (or peripheral arterial disease). And it is believed that nearly 5% of people age fifty and over are diagnosed with this disease which is somewhat more common in men than in women. Peripheral vascular disease (PVD) is a disease of the blood vessels (arteries and veins) positioned on the outer surface of the heart and brain. Although there are numerous causes of peripheral vascular disease, doctors often use the term when speaking of peripheral artery disease (peripheral arterial disease, PAD), a disease that develops when the arteries that supply blood to the internal organs, arms, and legs are entirely or to some extent blocked due to atherosclerosis.

- Heart healthy foods include: salmon, lemons, tomatoes, flaxseed (ground), oatmeal, black or kidney beans, almonds, walnuts, red wine, tuna, tofu, brown rice, soy milk, blueberries, carrots, spinach, broccoli, sweet potatoes, red bell peppers, asparagus, acorn squash, cantaloupe, papaya, and dark chocolate.

- Now let's review your food combinations: high starches should be eaten with low starches (vegetables); low starches (vegetables) with proteins. Eating high starches with protein is not a desirable combination because it can cause flatulence.

- Lettuce is composed of 95% water; therefore, as stated earlier, eat salads last during the meal so that its water content does not dilute digestive enzymes and to curve your appetite for desserts. Romaine lettuce is a better choice than iceberg.

- Remember to chew every bite at least 20 times. Don't rush through your meal and drink no more than 4 - 8 ounces of a beverage that has no ice. Then, as the Okinawans say, "hara hachi bu." Eat until you are 80% full. This is a great strategy to use to prevent overeating. For some, eating half the amount of food ordinarily consumed is a better strategy. Then enjoy dinner conversation and wait a few minutes before having a second serving because it takes your brain about 20 minutes to register that you are full. If you find that you are still hungry, eat another small portion and stop. My Grandfather (Papa) consumed food in this manner. I remember sitting at his dining room table and asking him why he ate such small portions (which was about half the amount most adults sitting at the table had on their plates). He replied, "You eat to nourish the body, not to fill up." Once he finished his meal, he would sit back in his chair and entertain others with dialogue that was very engaging. After some time had passed, if he was still hungry, he would serve himself a smaller portion; savor every bite; then sit back in his chair and compliment the cook. When asked if he was full, he replied, "No, I'm not full but I have eaten enough." Papa's physique was tall, lean and strong. He was a healthy man who lived to celebrate his 88th birthday.

- To indulge in wholesome dinner conversation does not mean that you discuss what happened on your job; what happened with the children at school; or your bills. Those issues can be stressful. Always give your food time to begin digesting without the tension.

- Dinner conversation should be enlightening and make the most of the time you spend with family and friends. There is something intimate about eating a meal together. You see a person in ways that you may not otherwise experience. There is a lot of vulnerability exposed when you eat with someone. Depending on whom you are sharing a meal with, dinner conversation could include topics ranging from thought provoking to silly discussions about travel, dating, books, relationships, movies, etc. A few examples of conversation starters would be: Tell me about the most beautiful place you have ever seen. Is science or art more essential to humanity? What was your most memorable meal ever? What historical time period would you most like to visit? Which personality trait has gotten you into the most trouble?

- The last person I asked about which personality trait had gotten him into the most trouble recited a laundry list of traits. I must admit that I was stunned by his response. Actually, I was almost in a state of shock. He explained his choices and we shared a wonderful moment of laughter.

- Laughter really is the best medicine. It not only makes you feel good but it is good for your health. It can reduce stress and boost your immune system. When laughing endorphins are released that suppress stress hormones. Laughter can also increase cells that destroy viruses and tumors. It lowers blood pressure as well. Find creative ways to add laughter to your life such as watching funny television shows; going to comedy clubs; and if all else fails, purchase joke books from your local book store. It is very important that you **LAUGH ABOUT SOMETHING EVERY DAY.**

- When eating out for dinner, many restaurants are very receptive about meeting your needs by using olive oil and soft margarine rather than butter; removing fat, skin, and certain herbs from dishes; and cooking entrees to order. Requests of this magnitude should be made when orders are placed, prior to the food being cooked.

- Order food in small portions and remember key words such as grilled, roasted, steamed, baked and poached. These entrees are healthier. When your order is a large serving of food, prepare a carryout box of half of the meal or share the entree with another person.

- Drink water or unsweetened green tea instead of soda.

- Beer, wine, and other alcoholic beverages. Calories from alcohol are stored as fat in the abdomen. Have you ever heard of "beer belly?"

- For optimum health benefits, women should have no more than one glass (4 oz.) of **RED WINE** per day and men two glasses (8 oz).

- Beer, white wine, and liquor do not have the health benefits of red wine.

- **People with certain health conditions should not consume alcoholic beverages at all. Talk to your doctor before taking the first drink. Find out if consuming beer, wine, or any other alcoholic beverage could be detrimental to YOUR health.**

- If bread is served prior to the meal and it is not whole grain or whole wheat, ask the waiter if they have any in the kitchen. If it is not available, you have a choice to make: either have no bread with your meal or eat only one piece because of the additional calorie intake. If you choose to eat only one piece of bread, serve yourself while the waiter remains at the table, then send the bread basket back to the kitchen.

- White bread and white rice have basically had all the nutrients processed out of them. They are considered empty calories. Brown rice is a healthier choice.

- Limit eating foods that are smoked; have cocktail sauce; or have been cooked in soy, teriyaki sauce, and au jus because of the high sodium content.

- In addition, you may want to limit or eliminate eating foods cooked on open BBQ grills that use charcoals as their heating source due to hydrocarbons absorbing into the food during the cooking process. Hydrocarbons have been linked to cancer. In fact, grilling 4 large stakes, 4 turkey cuts and 8 large sausages at the average 2-hour BBQ can release the same level of dioxins (chemicals known to increase the likelihood of cancer) as 220,000 cigarettes, according to a study by Robin de Bois.

- Gravies, salad dressings and sauces should be served on the side in order for you to control the amount you eat. Use them sparingly.

- Eat salads as the last entrée of your meal.

- Develop a habit of eating fresh fruit for dessert on a daily basis. Save sherbet and other desserts for special occasions such as birthdays, anniversaries, and holidays. Then indulge in only one serving.

- After the dinner meal, wait three hours before going to bed.

- Make sure you drink the remainder of your water at least thirty minutes before bedtime. Otherwise, you may find yourself having to use the bathroom during the night.

- Now the time has finally arrived for you to sit down and communicate about the events of the day with your significant others. Talk about what happened with the children at school; what happened at work; the bills, etc. If you have children, address their needs first. Once the children are settled, your focus should be on your significant other. The events of your day are the last thing you should mention. Then take care of the mundane day-to-day activities necessary to maintain a healthy household (i.e. pay the bills, clean the kitchen, wash clothes, etc.).

**What practices from the 6:30 PM hour do you need to incorporate in your evening routine in order to live a healthier lifestyle?**

- How will you achieve this goal?

- By when do you want to achieve this goal?

- What obstacles can be expected?

- What are the solutions to the obstacles?

## 7:00PM

- Reframe from doing anything that is mentally exhausting at least three hours before bedtime.

- At a minimum, once or twice a week you and your significant other should broaden your horizons and go on a date because whatever it took to get him (her) is the same thing that it's going to take to keep him (her). You have to work at keeping the fire and romance going in your relationship and dating is a vital part of that concept. Whether you have been together five months, five years, twenty-five years or more, dating can take your relationship to a different level.

- Visit an art gallery, museum, opera, a play, have dinner, go to church, a pro sports game, or even out for drinks in some quaint little shop or restaurant. The drinks don't have to be alcoholic. I know a husband and wife that rush out to a local coffee house every evening after putting the children to bed just to have a cup of coffee and share a few moments of down time together. As a different twist, my husband and I will meet at our favorite bookstore. We scurry to our preferred reading sections; scan all the shelves; and eventually pull two or three books. Then we meet each other in the café; order sandwiches and drinks; and find ourselves engrossed in the most relaxing, uninterrupted one hour of the day. With lifestyles as demanding as ours, it is almost impossible to find time to sit and leisurely read any kind of periodicals or books. Sometimes you will find the small, simple things in life so valuable.

- Whether you go out on a date for the evening or stay at home, immediately before settling in for bed, connect with your spouse again. Hug, snuggle, cuddle, caress, kiss, etc. Notice that all the actions that have been mentioned involve touching. That is very important, especially to women.

- The touching and physical connections may result in the two of you going as far as making love. That would be phenomenal. What better way do you know of releasing tension than making love to your spouse. It is similar to a workout. Believe it or not, depending on your weight, you can burn up to 200 calories while vigorously having sexual intercourse. After all, think about all the body parts being exercised in the process (arms, legs, thighs, buttocks, thorax, neck and even the circulatory system, to name a few). The more creative you are the more body parts can be involved. Then there is the breathtaking state of euphoria after your pleasure centers have been aroused by the release of endorphins and other chemicals in your brain. Now, I don't mean to stun you by any stretch of the imagination by making the following statement but let's face it. There is wonderful health benefits linked to being sexually active in the appropriate context. Couples that regularly (two or three times a week) engage in this type of intimacy are inclined to have more youthful appearances; and being more active in this area of your life will boost your immune system. The secret is to communicate, communicate, and communicate through all channels that have been made available to you. And men, try not to fall asleep immediately after you have made love. We realize that falling into a slumber state is a natural response for you due to the prolactin (induces a sleep state) being released in your body but a woman can not turn on and off the passion that quickly. Some things need to be massaged, caressed and taken pleasure in as the momentum changes and becomes suitable for both of you to find closure in the moment.

**What practices from the 7:00 PM hour do you need to incorporate in your evening routine in order to live a healthier lifestyle?**

- How will you achieve this goal?

- By when do you want to achieve this goal?

- What obstacles can be expected?

- What are the solutions to the obstacles?

## 8:00PM

- Take a warm bath or shower for thirty minutes roughly two hours before bedtime. The warmth of the water will cause a fall in your body temperature about two hours later that will make you sleepy.

- Ladies, after you get out of the shower, exfoliate your face at least two to three times a week unless you have oily skin. This should be done in order to remove the surface layer of dead cells on your face. Exfoliating more frequently may increase the chance of skin irritation, dryness or skin damage. After exfoliating, your skin should be radiant and fine lines appear less visible.

- Brush your teeth for a minimum of two minutes and floss.

- Flossing is imperative and should be done at least once a day. It not only removes food from between the teeth that regular brushing cannot reach but also eliminates plaque. If plaque is not removed your teeth decay and you are more susceptible to gum disease, cavities, and bad breath.

- **ONLY FLOSS THE TEETH YOU INTEND TO KEEP.**

- The probability of being diagnosed with gingivitis, periodontitis, tooth decay or oral cancer increases when a person smokes or uses smokeless tobacco.

- Using tobacco also contributes to bad breath and stains on your teeth.

- It is estimated that each year, Americans make about five hundred million visits to the dentists and over $102 billion dollars is spent on dental services.

- Discuss with your dentist how often you should schedule dental appointments. If you have a history of major dental work (fillings, crowns, bridge work, braces, etc.) you may have to visit the dentist regularly.

- Diabetics and smokers tend to have more gum disease than others; therefore, more frequent dental visits may become necessary.

- Likewise, individuals with suppressed immune systems (such as those with HIV) or receiving cancer treatment are also inclined to have dental problems; as a result, it is crucial that dental checkups are scheduled more frequently so as to sustain good oral wellness.

**What practices from the 8:00 PM hour do you need to incorporate in your evening routine in order to live a healthier lifestyle?**

- How will you achieve this goal?

- By when do you want to achieve this goal?

- What obstacles can be expected?

- What are the solutions to the obstacles?

## 10:00PM

- Avoid developing the habit of listening to the late night news. That may be challenging for you if you are like a lot of Americans that are excessive about the potential for crisis. However, it is better if you pass up filling your mind with those horrible stories before going to bed. Think about the majority of the stories you hear on the news. They are informing the public about something unpleasant that has happened. As far as the media is concerned, disaster sells. They are not really concerned about your mental state after absorbing that kind of information. Therefore, you are left with the task of choosing what kind of things you think on before going to sleep at night. Try to avert from exposing yourself to stimulus that is upsetting and/or depressing. Instead, quietly relax in your special place and allow your spirit to speak to you. Think on good things.

- To reduce the possibility of insomnia, avoid drinking caffeinated beverages in the evening; do not drink alcohol prior to going to bed; do not go to bed hungry; and resolve stress and anxiety before going to bed.

- Try to go to bed at the same time each night in order to develop a good sleep wake rhythmic pattern. Condition your mind to envision your bedroom as a place to make love and go to sleep. There is no other purpose.

- Never read, eat, watch television, or study in bed. These are activities that should be completed during the time you are awake and in any other room in the house except the bedroom.

- Now as you enter your slumber state, take pleasure in knowing that all that concerns you will be made perfect.

**What practices from the 10:00 PM hour do you need to incorporate in your bedtime routine in order to live a healthier lifestyle?**

- How will you achieve this goal?

- By when do you want to achieve this goal?

- What obstacles can be expected?

- What are the solutions to the obstacles?

# Note from the Author

*This book has depicted a person that chose to live a healthier lifestyle. In writing this book, my desire was that you envisioned yourself as that person. What life changes do you need to make? And what are you waiting for? Stop procrastinating because no excuse is acceptable. There is so much more that could have been added to these pages. However, many profound truths have been presented for your consideration. You have been given a choice between life and death. Choose life.*

# Additional Readings

*Student's life application Bible, New Living Translation, Tyndale House Publisher, Inc., Wheaton, Illinois, 1997.*
*http://www.medicinenet.com/kidney_stone/article.htm*

*http://www.americanheart.org/print_presenter.jhtml;jessionid=TLT12HCLA20CQFC*

*http://www.naturalnews.com/007133_grocery_warning_dangerous_foods.html*

*http://chaplaincare.navy.mil/selfhelp/stress.htm*

*http://www.medicinenet.com/osteoporosis/article.htm*

*http:// www.med.nyu.edu/patientcare/library/article.html?ChunkIID=164929*

*http://www.hsph.harvard.edu/nutritionsource/what-should- you-eat/protein/*

*http://emedicine.medscape.com/article/814774-overview*

*http://men.webmd.com/features/coffee-new-health-food*

*http://www.medicinenet.com/script/main/art.asp?articlekey=10358*

*http://www.medscape.com/viewarticle/721676*

http://www.medicinenet.com/running/article.htm.

http://leftofzen.com/brain-food/2008/01/04/

http://www.emedicinehealth.com/obesity_in_children/article_em.htm

http://www.medicinenet.com/aerobic_exercise/article.htm

http://www.webmd.com/sleep-disorders/guide/important-sleep-habits?page=2

http://www.medicinenet.com/cycling_biking_or_bicycling/article.htm

http://www.medicinenet.com/script/main/art.asp?articlekey= 59972&page=7#tock).

http://www.medicinenet.com/swimming/article.htm

http://www.medicinenet.com/high_blood_pressure/article.htm

http://www.medicinenet.com/ heart_ disease/article.htm

http://www.nlm.nih.gov/medlineplus/obesityinchildren.html

http://abcnews.go.com/GMA/Health/michelle-obama-childhood-obesity-initiative/story?id=9781473

http://www.medicinenet.com/cholesterol/article.htm

http://www.webmd.com/sleep-disorders/guide/sleep-requirements

http://www.medicinenet.com/smoking_and_quitting_smoking/article.htm

http://www.wordiq.com/definition/List_of_dance_style_categories

*http://www.nhlbisupport.com/bmi/bminojs.htm*

*http://www.webmd.com/fitness-exercise/features/exercise-at-your-desk*

# About The Author

*Dr. Elaine Lawrence Wynn's advice is as challenging as it is unambiguous. A certified Family Life Educator, Dr. Wynn specializes in the areas of interpersonal relationships, parenting, and healthy living. She has presented seminars around the country and internationally. Dr. Wynn is dedicated to building strength and adverting problems in individuals, couples, families, and parents through an educational approach – one relationship at a time. Her principles have helped thousands of individuals transform their lives. She is the author of Parenting With Ease and After the Affair. Dr. Wynn and her husband live in Atlanta, Georgia with their two sons.*